TOP FITNESS ADVICE

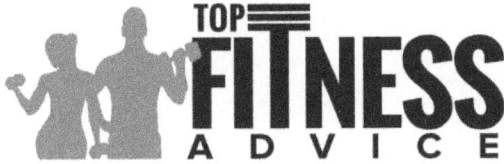

WEIGHT LOSS DIET

The #1 Rapid Weight Loss System for Busy People

LINDA WESTWOOD

ventureink
PUBLISHING

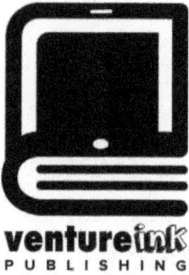

First published in 2016 by Venture Ink Publishing

For more information about the contents of this book or questions to the author, please contact Linda Westwood at linda@topfitnessadvice.com

Disclaimer

This book provides wellness management information in an informative and educational manner only, with information that is general in nature and that is not specific to you, the reader. The contents of this book are intended to assist you and other readers in your personal wellness efforts. Consult your physician regarding the applicability of any information provided in this book to you.

Nothing in this book should be construed as personal advice or diagnosis, and must not be used in this manner. The information provided about conditions is general in nature. This information does not cover all possible uses, actions, precautions, side-effects, or interactions of medicines, or medical procedures. The information in this book should not be considered as complete and does not cover all diseases, ailments, physical conditions, or their treatment.

You should consult with your physician before beginning any exercise, weight loss, or health care program. This book should not be used in place of a call or visit to a competent health-care professional. You should consult a health care professional before adopting any of the suggestions in this book or before drawing inferences from it.

Any decision regarding treatment and medication for your condition should be made with the advice and consultation of a qualified health care professional. If you have, or suspect you have, a health-care problem, then you should immediately contact a qualified health care professional for treatment.

No Warranties: The author and publisher don't guarantee or warrant the quality, accuracy, completeness, timeliness, appropriateness or suitability of the information in this book, or of any product or services referenced in this book.

The information in this book is provided on an "as is" basis and the author and publisher make no representations or warranties of any kind with respect to this information. This book may contain inaccuracies, typographical errors, or other errors.

Table of Contents

Would you prefer to listen to my book, rather than read it?

Download the audiobook version for free!

If you go to the special link below and sign up to Audible as a new customer, you can get the audiobook version of my book completely free.

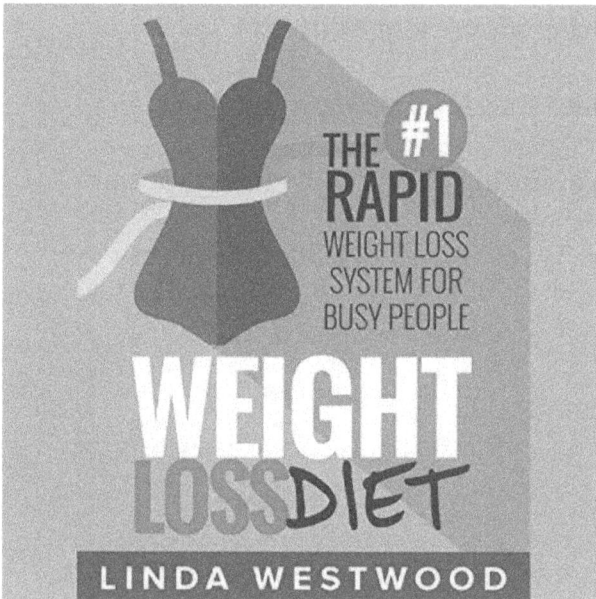

Go here to get your audiobook version for free:

TopFitnessAdvice.com/go/WeightLossDiet

Who is this book for?

In today's day and age, life keeps us busy. Hectically busy, in fact. Regardless of where you reside, we are all living in a fast-paced world. We rise early, stay at the office late and often feel like we don't have enough time to breathe, let alone eat right or exercise.

Instead, we stop at the nearest fast food joint on our way home from work; feed our children Happy Meals and Chinese food. Sure, we've wanted to lose that "winter belly" for two years now, but simply do not have the time.

And yes, this rings true for stay-at-home mom's just as it does for the working mother or father – their grind is taking care of house and home, transporting children to and from soccer practice, gymnastic or football, ensuring they do their homework accurately and on time. The list goes on.

The point is: no matter who you are, where you live or what you do for a living, many of us find it difficult to find enough time in the day to take care of our body, nourishing it with whole, healthy food and exercising regularly.

And because of that, dieting or losing weight has become a task—one that is much harder than our day to day. To many of us, losing weight has become *impossible*.

Does any of this sound familiar? If so, this book is for you. The mother. The father. The businesswoman. The businessman. The freelancer. The entrepreneur. This book is for anyone and *everyone* who wants to make a positive change toward health in their life.

You'll be amazed to learn that in as little as thirty minutes (10 minutes, three times a day), you can begin to reach your diet and fitness goal. It's not impossible and that change is right around the corner.

What will this book teach you?

This fast-paced read is going to put each and every one of you on the fast track to dieting and exercise success. You will learn how to seamlessly implement simple techniques on a regular basis to keep yourself motivated and focused on the goal at hand.

Regardless of whether you want to lose 5, 10, 50 or 100 pounds, you can meet your goal in a matter of weeks (days, even) by making a few adjustments to your routine and mindset.

Even if you work more than 70 hours a week you can squeeze some seriously healthy habits into even the busiest of schedules.

Many people have a daily routine that is just that: *routine.* Sure, you wake up early, get to the office early and stay late, but what about your body?

You are fueling yourself with fast food, energy drinks and unhealthy carbs to keep yourself moving when in actuality, fueling yourself with a healthy alternative will give you much more energy.

I know, I know. All of this is well and good, but it's a million times easier to grab a pre-packaged breakfast sandwich than it is to make a veggie scramble, right?

Well if you *plan* ahead, you will be able to grab that veggie scramble just as fast (if not faster) than that fat-and-carb-filled breakfast sandwich.

Routine is about sticking to schedules in order to manage our life a little better, so within this book you will learn how to **open your mind, stay determined and implement a healthy routine** – a routine that will change your life for the better, inside and out.

Introduction

Life. Life is chaotic, isn't it? When we were teenagers, we couldn't wait to be an adult, to manage our own life and do as we please. No more curfews, rules or regulations. Nope, as an adult we get to live it up: we can stay up late, sleep in for as long as we want, eat whatever junk food we'd like and have cereal for dinner every single day of the week.

Well, at least until we are married with children. *Maybe.*

If your mother was anything like mine, junk food didn't exist in our house. It would rot our teeth and our minds. We didn't even eat fast food. My mom's idea of fast food was using premade pizza crust, adding mozzarella and pepperoni, and then tossing it in the oven. That's the extent of fast food that was experienced in my childhood home.

The only time I ate a McDonald's Cheeseburger Happy Meal was when I would spend the night at my best friend's house. Both parents worked full-time jobs and it was much easier for them to pick up fast food than to prepare something at home. I thought my friend was the luckiest kid alive but once I hit adulthood, I understood.

And when I say adulthood, I mean after college once I hit the workforce. On that very day my world changed forever. What I realized was: *I don't have any time!*

I didn't have time for anything. It was go-go-go and with that, fast food became my go-to. I did have some free weights at home that I used, but aside from that – for years I didn't know what cardio or healthy eating was. It just wasn't part of my *routine*. It couldn't be if I wanted to prove to my boss that I was worth my first promotion and then the next.

Sound familiar? See, all of the above really isn't about me. It's about *us* as human beings in the 21st century. This is equally true for moms and dads, stockbrokers, attorneys, doctors, bakers, chefs and even baggers at your local grocer. Though the day job might be different, learning to manage time and implement healthy habits is the same for all of us.

Now, before we can successfully achieve our wellness and weight loss goals, we need to tackle the most difficult aspect of our existence—our mind and body. When first adjusting your daily routine, you will find that your mind and body has a large role in that change, and whether or not you will stick with the plan or give up.

Motivation and determination regarding dieting and health do not come easy. If it did, you wouldn't be looking for a change in your life and it's not likely that you'd be reading this book. The mind is a powerful thing; even the subconscious mind. A positive mindset goes a long way, especially within the realm of health, dieting and fitness.

In Chapter One you will learn to crush negative vibes and replace them with something positive and enlightening. Today is a new day and marks the first day of the rest of your life. Today you will venture off on a diet and wellness journey that will change your hectic life for the better so that you can live a fuller, happy, healthier *you*.

Chapter One

Mind & Body

As mentioned in the Introduction, the key to a successful change of routine—dieting or losing weight, in particular—is a positive mindset or a switch in limited thinking.

When we are wrapped up in our current life or situation, we often think that there's *no possible way* to make a change, especially if it requires some *more* of your time. I mean, you barely have enough time to breathe, how on Earth could you exercise or make a home cooked meal?

It might not seem possible, but the power of positive thinking goes a long way. Not only will you feel empowered, it is a significant factor in your weight loss goals.

At the same time, however, it is not uncommon to experience self-doubt as you begin your journey especially when you do something 'you're not supposed to'.

You know, beating yourself up every time you eat the wrong foods, constantly focusing on what you cannot eat, and approaching your new exercise regimen with dread instead of excitement.

These feelings of self-doubt are very common but the truth is that changing your dieting and eating habits doesn't need to be so restricting. The typical dieting world is full of the 'All or Nothing' scenario, making it far too difficult for *most* people to stick with the plan let alone someone who doesn't have much free time as it is.

Luckily, this doesn't have to be the case because changing your diet and eating habits doesn't need to be restricting. You don't need to resort to eating rice cakes and carrots, drinking Slim Fast or nutritional bars that really aren't all that nutritious in the first place. By implementing a new schedule and healthier alternatives, you can essentially eat all of your favorite foods.

Well, except McDonald's or Taco Bell.

You might be thinking to yourself, *'All of this sounds great but how do I keep myself motivated or positive like that?'*

Yes, it will take some practice but there are a few strategies that you can use to increase your positive thinking *today.*

You'll find that once you adopt a positive mindset things will start falling into place and good things will come to fruition— including shedding those pounds. The 'Law of Attraction' starts with attitude.

Six Strategies to Develop a Positive Mindset

1. *There's Nothing Like the Present.*

Living in the moment is much easier than it sounds. We have all been through difficult things in life, all very different from one another, but difficult just the same.

As human beings it's very common to think about the past.

As Mark Twain once said, 'I've been through terrible things in my life, some of which actually happened.' This rings true for all of us because at one point or another, we are letting our past control us.

We focus on what we did or didn't do, how we shouldn't have had that whole pizza, that cheeseburger or whatever else it might have been. We focus on the potential of something negative or worrisome happening for days on end, only for it to not happen at all.

Anxiety. Focusing on the negative or the past keeps us from moving forward. If we can learn how to live in the present, our mind will be centered and in a positive space.

2. *The Use of Positive Language, Canceling Out Negative Vibes*

'I can't stand my job.'

'Why does it always have to rain on my day off?'

'If I would get some more help around here, I would have time to go to the gym.'

If you give it some thought, you'd be surprised how often our language is filled with negativity. It's only natural for us to get down in the dumps on occasion, but if we are not happy with our self-image or wellness goals these thoughts can become all too consuming.

Using negative language can only bring forth doubt, making it extremely difficult for us to accomplish our goals—especially diet or weight loss goals. Our words are shaped by our thoughts, so if you start using positive language over negative, you will begin to think more positively and achieve positive results.

I'm sure you're thinking that this has to be more difficult than I'm making it out to be, but there are actually quite a few techniques that I've used over the years—techniques that work as good as magic.

Grab yourself a notebook that you can use as your 'Negative Thought Squasher' or whatever you'd like to call it.

What you'll do with this notebook is write down any negative thoughts you've had throughout the day. If you're lacking willpower and simply cannot just squash those cravings, write it down.

Writing these negative thoughts or emotions down will essentially be acknowledging them. And guess what? By acknowledging those negative emotions, they will start having less power on you. You can then make a conscious effort to transform your thoughts, providing you with optimal results.

3. *Learn to Accept that Things Aren't Perfect.*

Yes, we want them to be perfect but there's no such thing as perfect. While it might be frustrating for us to see that our neighbor, friend or colleague has lost more weight in two weeks than you have in a year, everyone is different and we are perfectly imperfect.

If you can stick with that positive outlook, you will have the ability to just accept things as they are and trust the process. Sure, it might take you a while longer than your sister or brother to reach your weight loss and fitness goals, but you're steadily losing weight and it will happen. The important thing to remember is that it will happen, it is happening and you're dedicated to the process.

You're dedicated to this change in your routine—a change that will positively change your life for the better.

4. *Stick with Supportive People*

No one needs a Debbie Downer in their life, particularly when they are focused on staying MOTIVATED. While it's understandable that there is a Debbie Downer or two in every group, it's best to avoid them like the plague. Being mixed up with those negative vibes is just as difficult as sitting next to someone smoking a cigarette when you are trying to quit. It's not possible.

This doesn't mean that you need to shun your family or friends who just so happen to fit in the Debbie Downer category; it just means that you need to predominantly stick with positive, supportive folks.

Meetup.com and other online support or chat groups are fantastic for staying motivated and mixing with likeminded individuals who are after a similar goal. The more you stay with positive thinking individuals, the more positive you will begin to think/feel as well. Laughter is the best medicine and it's an incredible stress-reducer.

5. *Set Manageable Goals*

We are going to discuss this later in this book, but it needs to be mentioned here, especially because setting manageable goals has a lot to do with our mindset.

For instance, if we set unrealistic weight loss goals, try to exist on an extremely low-calorie diet or try to set an unattainable number for weekly weight loss goals, you are setting yourself up for failure.

And after week one and not reaching that '5 pound goal', you could very well throw in the towel and your mindset will revert back to the negative, 'There's no way I'm ever going to lose weight' mindset.

Setting manageable goals are imperative to fostering positive thinking.

6. *Comedy – Laughter as Medicine.*

Going to a comedy show, movie or watching one at home can be as good as medicine. While the point of this book is you learning how to shed pounds, lose weight and adopt a healthier life despite your hectic schedule, fitting in some time to laugh is imperative. Laughter is medicine—it has been proven to reduce stress, providing a full-on workout for muscles, unleashing a rush of stress-shattering endorphins.

It might seem odd, but the truth is that our bodies can't distinguish between real and fake laughter. Even fake laughter will have a positive impact on your day-to-day life. A sense of humor is not required, just a good ol' hearty laugh.

You'll find that once you start implementing the above six strategies, your life will begin to transform for the better. Keeping a positive mindset will help you push forward and truly benefit from this powerful life change.

In Chapter Two we are going to talk about diving in to your new routine...but with baby steps. It's not necessary to dive in head first and not come up for air. It's important that we drop that 'All or Nothing' mentality and trust the process.

If you've been the 'All or Nothing' kind of person in the past, it's time to drop that madness and stop swinging back and forth.

Discover Scientifically-Proven "Shortcuts" & "Hacks" to Lose Weight FASTER (With Very Little Effort)

For this month only, you can get Linda's best-selling & most popular book absolutely free – *Weight Loss Secrets You NEED to Know*.

Get Your FREE Copy Here:
TopFitnessAdvice.com/Bonus

Discover scientifically-proven tips to help you lose weight faster and easier than ever before. With this book, readers were able to improve their weight loss results and fitness levels. So, it's highly recommended that you get this book, especially while it's free!

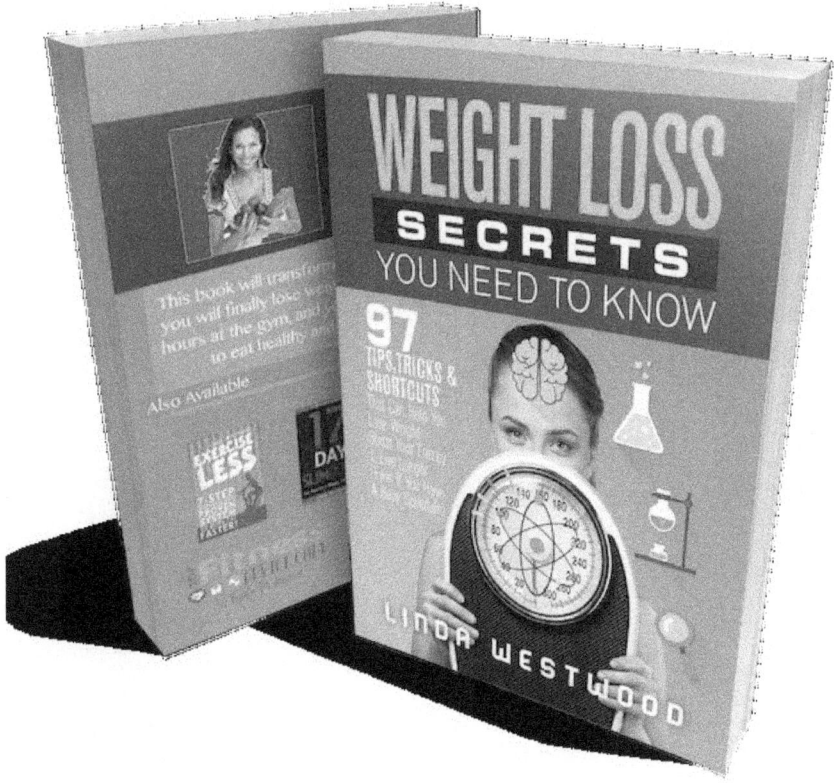

Get Your FREE Copy Here:

TopFitnessAdvice.com/Bonus

Chapter Two

But First...Baby Steps

Today is the first day of the rest of your life.

It's a completely natural feeling to want to dive in head first to a new dieting plan, but what makes *our process* different is that we aren't really on a specific diet plan per se, we are creating a new routine that delivers results. A *routine* that becomes a constant force in our hectic daily life.

In the 21st Century there are a gazillion diets that swamp the market. There is Paleo, Weight Watchers, Low Carb, Pescatarian, Body for Life, Nutrisystem, Slim Fast, South Beach Diet, the Atkins Diet and more. It's a cluttered industry and everyone seems to know the *right way* to lose weight.

But somehow, with your chaotic schedule, you just can't seem to make it happen. You've tried it all, so what gives?

There are a couple different reasons this happens:

First, it's a very common thing to put too much pressure on ourselves regarding our diet or weight loss plan and when we don't shed the pounds we thought we would within a week, we throw in the towel.

Secondly, we often don't fully commit to the possibility of losing weight and making that possibility a *reality*. That commitment is a big reason why we make or break things, especially when it comes to routine and a life-change for the better.

Committing to a change in routine is sometimes very difficult, especially when we have lived a certain way for months or years on end. But by taking baby steps, it can and *will happen*. Losing weight is about energy balance, not about counting calories or eating pre-made foods for weight loss.

In addition to the above, our body is a working organism and can sometimes work against us in this game called Life—especially when it comes to weight loss. Before we dive into the remainder of the book and discuss how you can meet your weight loss goals, I want to talk about a few reasons why people do not achieve their desired weight loss—outside of blaming their busy schedule.

For instance, maybe in the past you have had success with losing weight, without putting in much effort. Yippee!! Maybe you ate the same foods, but exercised a bit more and managed to lose ten pounds. But then suddenly the weight loss slowed down or stopped all together.

Bummer. This can be a motivation crusher. You were stoked when you lost those first six pounds and within a week you're back to your old mindset.

Sometimes this happens and I want to briefly discuss some of the common reasons you are not managing to lose weight. Gaining this knowledge will allow you to move forward, breaking through the plateau and getting things moving again.

Ten Common Reasons You're Not Losing Weight

1. You're Losing Weight Without Realizing It.

Oddly enough, this happens more often then you'd think. Maybe you jump on the scale each morning only to find that you're steady and those numbers haven't budged for a few days or even a few weeks. While this is discouraging, try to keep in mind that this doesn't mean you aren't losing fat.

The unfortunate fact is that body weight tends to fluctuate by a few pounds depending on how much water you drink and on the type of food you're eating. Later I will talk about the effect processed foods have on our body, but this can be a big issue when it comes to shedding those pounds.

Additionally, if you're exercising to lose weight, you could be gaining muscle as you lose fat. If this is the case, you're actually on the right track because you want to lose fat, not just weight. Also, how well your clothing fits can be very telling.

2. You're Not Drinking Enough COLD Water.

We all know that water equals life and that we need to drink at least 2 liters (or a half gallon) of water each day, but did you know that this life water can actually help you lose weight?

Cold water, that is. When you drink cold water, your body uses extra calories to warm the water to body temperature.

In a recent 12-week weight loss study, people who drank 17 ounces of cold water 30 minutes before meals lost 44% more eight.

In addition to the study, drinking water has also been known to boost the amount of calories burned by 24-30% over a period of one and a half hours.

What does this mean? Drink more water!

3. *You Are Not Eating Enough* WHOLE FOODS.

We are going to talk more about this throughout the book, but open the trash can and throw out the processed foods and begin a diet rich in whole foods. The quality of your food is just as important as quantity.

High quality foods can regulate your appetite because they tend to be more filling than their processed equivalents.

This means that you should stick to whole, single-ingredient foods as often as possible, steering clear of any processed foods that are labeled as being health foods. They might have the word 'health' in them, but they aren't actually that healthy at all. AND, they won't help you shed the pounds.

4. *Protein, Protein, Protein.*

It doesn't matter if you're eating lean meats, tofu, beans or seafood; protein is one of the most important nutrients for losing weight. In fact, eating protein at 30% calories can boost your metabolism by 80 to even 100 calories per day, automatically making you eat several hundred fewer calories per day.

Additionally, eating protein can reduce cravings and desires for snacking. We all know how difficult it is to toss the Heluva Good Dip out the window, but that sucker isn't doing you any good. (Yeah, yeah...we know).

For those of you who eat breakfast, this is the best meal of the day to load up on protein. High-protein breakfasts will help curb your hunger throughout the day, ensuring you have fewer unhealthy snacks and fewer cravings throughout the day.

For those of you who eat a solid portion of protein will help prevent metabolic slowdown—a common side effect of losing weight. It will also help to prevent weight regain, assisting you in staying within your preferred weight range.

5. *You're Drinking Sugar.*

I know it's hard to avoid some days because sugar-filled beverages line the shelves, including those energy drinks that we sometimes (ahem, I mean always) consume in order to manage our hectic lifestyle. They have become the norm and anyone who's anyone drinks a Red bull and Monster to stay alert and alive. Black coffee just doesn't cut it.

You'd be surprised that the list of sugary drinks isn't just limited to drinks like Monster, Red bull, Coke and Pepsi; it also applies to the "healthier" alternatives the market tries to persuade you with such as Vitamin Water. Vitamin Water is actually packed full of sugar even though it prides itself on being "enhanced" water.

6. *You Binge Eat...And Yes, It's Possible to Binge on Healthy Foods.*

When people dive in and establish that "all or nothing" mentality, a common side effect of this type of dieting (or extreme dieting), is binge eating. Most people would think of binge eating as eating unhealthy food such as sweets, ice cream and other fats.

However, binge eating is as simple as rapidly eating large amounts of food—much more than your body needs.

Despite what you'd think, binge eating is a problem for many dieters. And while some might binge on junk food, others will binge on relatively healthy foods including nuts, nut butters, dark chocolate, cheese and so on.

While something might be healthy, calories still count and very much exist.

7. *Calories, Count.*

Just as I mentioned above, calories count. Even if you don't "binge" eat healthy food, a large portion of people who have an issue with losing weight (or losing as much as they want, at least) are eating too many calories.

Counting calories can be annoying sometimes, I know, but if you aren't losing weight, it's important that you weigh your food and track you calories for a while.

It doesn't have to be long-term, but maybe a week. A week will give you solid looks into your day-to-day eating habits and how many calories you're actually consuming.

With the technological era we live in there are a variety of resources that can be helpful in tracking calories including **Food Tracker**.

In addition to ensuring that you're staying on track regarding your calorie intake, tracking your food is also important if you're trying to reach a certain nutrient goal (i.e. getting a % of your calories from protein).

Again, keeping track of your calories isn't something that you need to do for the rest of your life.

A few days to a week to get a feel for what you should be eating is all that's necessary.

8. *Cardio is Good for Your Heart and for A Balanced Life.*

I know, I know...this book is all about dieting and losing weight on a hectic schedule, so I'm sure you're wondering how the heck you could even consider implementing cardio in your daily routine. Between rush hour and soccer, you don't have a second to yourself. A jog? Hmm.

We will talk about adjusting your routine to allow some time for exercise a little later on in this book. For now, I simply want to mention that cardio is one of the most effective ways to improve your overall health. Not only that, if you're really want to burn belly fat and that harmful "visceral" fat that builds up around organs causing disease, cardio is a one-stop-shop, giving you everything you need.

9. *Insomniac Nation.*

Insomniac Nation sounds like an 80's rock band, but in reality, our nation and nations around the world are made up of insomniacs. We work, work, work and hit the grind hard, getting up early and staying at the office late. We are a world of addicts and while most people won't see being addicted to work as a "bad" thing, we are not getting enough sleep.

Good, solid sleep is one of the most important things to consider for your physical and mental health, not to mention your weight. Many studies have shown that poor sleep is one of the single biggest risk factors for obesity. Adults and children with poor sleep have a 55% and 89% greater risk of becoming obese.

While some of us can manage our day-to-day life with just four hours of sleep, the National Sleep Foundation recommends 7-9 hours of sleep each night (for an adult).

10.   *Everyone loves carbs, but carbs don't love us back.*

We all know this, right? This doesn't necessarily mean that you need to cut carbs out completely, but cutting back is important. In short-term studies, this type of diet has been shown to cause up to 3 times as much weight loss as the standard low-fat diet. In addition to weight loss, minimizing your carb intake can lead to improvements in triglycerides, blood sugar and HDL cholesterol.

While there are a few other reasons why people might not be losing weight, the details noted above are some of the most common. We will talk more about this throughout the remaining chapters.

Before going onto the next chapter where we will talk about the importance of squeezing in some extra movement throughout your day, I want to quickly discuss a few baby steps that you can tackle when preparing for your *new* daily routine.

Changing Your Routine Little by Little

When you're making a positive change in order to achieve your weight loss goals, one of the first steps you need to take is to toss out all the garbage in your cabinets and refrigerator. If you don't want to waste all that processed food, you can always donate it to a shelter or soup kitchen. Once it's out of your kitchen, consider it out of your life.

Today is the first day of the rest of your life. This speaks volumes. Today, you are going to dispose of convenience foods and ready-made meals such microwaveable dinners, frozen dinners and breaded frozen meats (i.e. chicken nuggets, tenders, fish), canned food, ramen noodles, frozen pizza and so on. Food processing techniques include freezing, canning, baking, drying and pasteurizing products.

Frozen veggies and fruit are okay, of course. And it's not the end of the world if you grab some pre-bagged spinach or veggies as they are minimally processed.

Once you've managed to rid your life of processed goods, it's time to make a weekly grocery list. Now, we all know that it's a natural tendency to go out and buy all "fat free" or "low carb" options, but the truth is that *whole foods* are the way to go.

Making meal choices that are packed with lots of fruits, vegetables, eggs, seafood and meat—and that are minimally processed—is one of the best life changes you can make. While it's great to eat less fat, products that are listed as "fat free" are often packed with other no-nos.

In addition to being awesome for your body, this fresh diet will eliminate your want of processed foods—meaning boxed meals, breakfast bars, etc.

Processed foods came about in the 1950's and 60's and were broadcasted everywhere. They made our life easier, right? Not only could we have a "home cooked meal" in under ten minutes, we could enjoy a variety of food that was created with time management in mind.

While processed food was seen as exciting back then (because it was *new),* since the 1960's, the United States has tripled its obesity rate. **Yes, tripled!** And more than that, type 2 diabetes in children has increased by more than 30% and seven out of ten adults are overweight.

Many people with a hectic schedule think that the only way they can fuel their body is by consuming pre-packaged breakfast bars and other quick-foods, but you can eliminate this problem by weekend meal-prep, pre-making go-to meals that are made from whole foods, instead of their processed counterpart.

For example, instead of grabbing a breakfast or protein bar for an early morning pick me up; you can nuke a couple egg muffins that you made over the weekend. It's simple to make 10 or more for the week, keeping two days' worth in the fridge and then tossing the others in the freezer until the night before. That way in the morning all you need to do is toss them in the microwave for 30 seconds and run out the door. Simple as that.

And these "muffins" are easy to make and take less than 30 minutes from start to finish. Not only that, they will fill you up for hours, making it less likely for you to grab bagged snacks.

Meal prep over the weekend might take a few hours, but it ensures that your weekly daytime (breakfast and lunch) meals are easy. By making this change, tossing out processed foods and staying dedicated to health(ier) alternatives, you will find that your cravings for the bad stuff will fade away.

In the next chapter we are going to discuss the importance of movement and how adding just thirty minutes of exercise throughout your day can make a world of difference to your weight loss efforts. Sure, you're busy, but I want to disclose the many ways that you can add mini-workouts to your day without much effort.

I hope that you are enjoying this book so far, and if you could spare 30 seconds, I would greatly appreciate you leaving a review on Amazon.com.

Chapter Three

Movement Matters

You're too busy to watch your favorite television show, so how on Earth could you possibly add movement or exercise to your day? It's impossible, right? Most people assume that they need to dedicate more than an hour a day to solid exercise in order to actually lose weight but this couldn't be further from the truth.

A recent study has shown that just thirty minutes of exercise per day might be the golden number. And better yet, it doesn't have to be all at one time. This means that you can actually add mini-workouts throughout your day to equal thirty minutes.

Sounds more manageable, eh?

Within this study researchers found that men who exercised hard enough to sweat for a total of thirty minutes a day lost an average of eight to nine pounds over a three-month period, compared to an average weight loss of six pounds among men who worked out for 60 minutes or more a day.

According to Mads Rosenkilde, a PhD student at the University of Copenhagen, part of the reason for this weight loss success was because those who found 30 minutes of exercise a day doable actually had the desire (and energy) for additional exercise or physical activity.

While it's imperative to work up a sweat at least 30 minutes a day, this is actually quite simple and doesn't require you to make a trip to the gym (because sometimes—most days—we don't have the time for that).

I know what you're thinking...." *yeah, right!"* But there are actually some very simply ways to add exercise into your day even when you have zero time. Stolen moments throughout your day add up and will help you shed those pounds in no time.

Listed below are a variety of ways that you can add at least 30 minutes of workout magic throughout your day regardless of whether you're at home, the office, watching TV with the kids, while traveling (on a business trip) and more.

So, let's get to it.

20 Ways to Sneak in Mini-Workouts Throughout Your Day

1. If you're at home, when you go outside to pick up your morning newspaper (or mail), take a brisk five-minute walk up the street in one direction and then back to your place. You might think that you'll look hilarious taking a quick jaunt in your pajamas, but it's an easy addition to your busy day.

2. Did you know that a 150-pound woman can burn **90 calories** in just *one* 10-minute jumping jack session? Yes, jumping jacks can burn calories quite easily—you

can do jumping jacks at home or at the office (in between meetings).

3. If you're waiting for a pot of water to boil or food to cook through for dinner, do a set of ten (or more) easy peasy standing push-ups.

   All you need to do is stand at an arm's length from the kitchen counter and then push your arms against the counter. Inhale and then in one movement, press your body toward the counter as if you're doing a regular push-up. That's it.

4. If you have children, try to set aside some time after dinner for play. This could be shooting some hoops, playing tag, football or maybe even riding bikes as a family. Not only will this give your kids some great lasting memories, you will get in some solid calorie kicking exercise.

5. Does your child play soccer, take karate, voice lessons or gymnastics? If you find yourself waiting for your children to finish their extracurricular activity, walk around the block a few times. As you begin to exercise more regularly, bring your sneakers and add one to two minutes of jogging to those walks.

6. Going to the playground with your kids? Bring a ball and play with your kids.

7. If you live in the city or in close proximity to your work opt to walk or ride your bike to the office. If you bike,

say, a few miles every day, you will begin to see results in no time.

8. Office lunch meetings? Opt to dine out at a restaurant that is a little bit out of your way. Choose to walk (or bike), not drive.

9. If your afternoon business meeting is in another building, take some time after the scheduled meeting to sneak in an afternoon power walk.

10. It might seem silly, but if your office has staircases, use them to your advantage and climb stairs on your lunch hour. It doesn't have to be long—5 to 10 minutes of stair climbing will do the trick.

11. Elevator abs has never been more fun and what's awesome is that you can strengthen your core, even in a packed elevator. All you need to do is practice standing with your feet parallel and your knees relaxed.

12. Music therapy. When you're doing laundry or cleaning house, turn on Spotify and dance like no one is watching (because they aren't).

13. If you're heading out on a business trip, remember to bring your sneakers. You can manage a quick speed walk in your day somewhere. Worst case, do a series of jumping jacks three times a day to hit your 30-minute exercise mark.

14. Pick up some free weights and keep them somewhere in your living room or bedroom. Do some easy lifts in the morning while you're getting ready for your day and before bed.

15. Taking a red-eye out or morning flight for a business meeting? Be sure to avoid the "moving carpets" that assist travelers in transporting from concourse to concourse. Walk around as much as possible.

16. Do some standing crunches during your lunch break to work your abdominal area.

17. Order a resistance band and bring it to the office to use on your lunch break or during any "free time" you might have throughout the day. A few minutes here or there can really add up.

18. Switch to an adjustable standing desk that you can transition from a traditional desk to standing throughout the day. Standing burns more calories than sitting, but when you do sit at your desk try to make sure that you have good posture and that your back is properly supported.

19. Stretch your calves during elevator rides (if you're alone, of course).

20. Book your hotel room on the fifth floor and skip the elevators.

As you can see, there are quite a few ways that you can sneak in some mini-exercises throughout your day, regardless of how busy or hectic your schedule is.

In many ways adding as little as two 30-second "bursts" of high intensity exercise like jumping jacks or sprinting, or multiple mini-workouts throughout your day can provide more opportunities for weight loss over one long workout per day (that many of us simply do not have time for).

The cool thing about implementing a mini-workout program throughout the day is that the exercise is done for about two to three minutes, six to eight times per day.

For those of you who are home during the day, you could implement mini-workouts that consist of three 10-minute workouts. Everyone is different, so it's important for you to figure out which type of regimen will be ideal for your lifestyle.

Some of you might be thinking that the mini-exercises mentioned above sound more than *ridiculous*, but you'd be surprised just how simple they will be to implement.

And the great thing about adding exercise to your daily routine is that there are a ton of other reasons exercise can and will benefit your life, more so than just weight loss.

Once you begin implementing these mini-exercises you will find that you will have a boost in mood and energy. Not only that, you will able to sleep much more sound and have less stress, anxiety and/or depression.

As you begin exercising it's important to be kind to yourself. Don't put far out expectations on yourself and remember self-compassion is important. Keeping your expectations reasonable will increase the likelihood that you will succeed at any endeavor—including weight loss!

Don't overthink your weight loss endeavors, either. Remember that everyone is at a different fitness level so it's completely okay if you're tired after your first day. Soon enough you will fly through each workout with ease and with that, you will also find that your willpower will increase considerably.

Remember, however, that you didn't get out of shape overnight which also means that your body isn't going to transform after a day, either. That said, keep that positive mindset in check and try not to be discouraged by what you can do or how far you have to go to shed the 30 to 50 pounds you want to lose. Consistency is key and as you continue to work these mini-workouts throughout your day physical payoff will come.

In addition to these mini-workouts you can make exercise fun with your family and friends. If you have a family, significant other or children, you can work together as a team to make exercise fun, creating goals that you can achieve together.

Today's world is driven by technology, more than half of children are not enthusiastically active on a regular basis. Instead we are chilling out in front of the TV watching Netflix or Hulu, or playing our favorite video game. And unfortunately, inactive children often grow into sedentary adults.

Sad, but true.

However, implementing a family fitness regimen will not only help build a bond with your loved ones, it will mesh seamlessly with your weight loss goals and break the '*I have no time to exercise!*' pattern that plagues so many of us.

If you don't have time throughout your day to exercise a total of 30 minutes, you can add snippets of exercise during your family time. And if you make this a family fun time you can change up the way you're exercising regularly to make things exciting—biking, skating, playing ball, nightly walks, jogs etc.

One of my closest friends, for example, started jogging with her 11-year-old daughter every night or at least every other night. Her daughter started becoming more interested in running and joined this club called "Girls on the Run" where she started running three miles regularly.

I know three miles is a lot for most of us, but my friend used this mobile app called 'Couch to 5k' which trained her for her first 5k where she ran side-by-side with her daughter. Never did she think she would run that distance, but within one month it was possible. And guess what? She became so much closer to her daughter, making this a regular routine for 'mommy/daughter' time *and* she lost 30 pounds!

If you simply don't have time for extra daily exercise outings with your family, try to make it a weekend thing—something to look forward to after a long, tiring week. Your family will thank you, and so will your body.

Influence is everything and as you start these little routines throughout the day and with your loved ones, your mind will shift and exercise will become second nature. Soon enough, you won't think about it as 'exercise' because it will become a way of life.

Now that we've talked about mindset and adding exercise to your daily routine, in the next chapter I want to talk about adding a healthy morning juice regimen to your life. Not only is juicing easy, it will reboot your system and make it much less likely for you to grab sweets or unhealthy eats. It's also a much better alternative than grabbing a breakfast bar, pop tart or highly processed (yet oh so yummy, I know) breakfast sandwich.

Once again, thank you for reading this book, and I hope you're getting a lot of valuable information. I would greatly appreciate it if you could take 30 seconds to leave me a review for this book on Amazon.com.

Enjoying this book?

Check out my other best sellers!

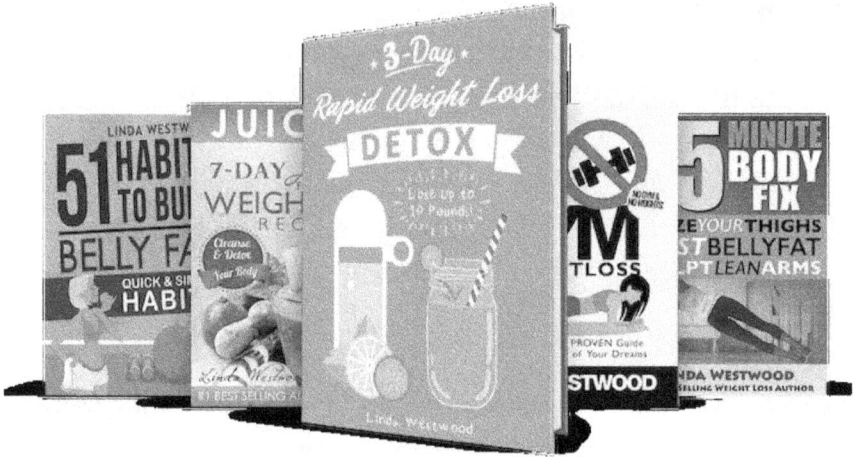

Chapter Four

Two Minute Morning Juice

Anyone who's anyone has heard of juicing or smoothies these days. Sure, they are all the rave—but for good reason. Before I get into how juicing will help with your weight loss efforts, there are a million other ways that a morning juice can positively affect your everyday life.

Think about all of the goodness that goes into a morning juice. Sure, you can mix it up and create different recipes, but there are a few must-haves within every juice or health shake:

1. Greens (kale, baby spinach, chards, etc.)

2. Veggies (avocado, carrots, broccoli, celery, etc.)

3. Fruit (strawberries, blueberries, banana, mango etc.)

4. Protein powder (optional)

5. Almond milk (optional)

Lots of people, maybe even you, look at the list above and think, '*Yuck! There's no way in hell I'm drinking that!*' But the weird thing is that these juices actually taste good. While greens can be bitter, the fruit offsets that bitterness and adds the perfect amount of sweet.

In addition to being a quick and easy breakfast choice, juicing has the power to improve your energy levels as well as provide many other physical and mental benefits including weight loss, improved digestion, reduced appetite, improved skin appearance and more.

When your mind and body is used to packing in all of that processed food, a reboot (by juicing regularly) can essentially turn your lifestyle around. You'll find that in a matter of days you will no longer crave sweets, chips or any other go-to snacks. Instead you will more than likely crave fruits, vegetables and healthy meal options.

While, yes, you have a busy lifestyle—a busy lifestyle doesn't mean that you need to keep getting bogged down by unhealthy lifestyle choices. Dropping the sugar and processed foods will make a world of difference, and it doesn't hurt to limit your caffeine and alcohol intake.

Believe me, I love my coffee and whiskey (or red wine) just as much as the rest of you but moderation will help knock off those pounds in a jiffy. Yes, I said jiffy. You'd be surprised how fast you will lose weight by limiting your alcohol intake, especially if you're someone who drinks regularly to 'let off steam.'

A 2010 review published in *Physiology and Behavior* noted that drinking alcohol before or during meals tends to increase the number of calories one consumes during a meal.

Thus, not drinking alcohol around meals can help you cut down calories from your diet. Minimizing your fat intake can also make a difference as alcohol calories seem to be most likely to affect weight in people who don't drink or who eat a high-fat diet.

Now, back to juicing. When you set off to change your daily routine on this weight loss venture it is vital to note that a daily juice can give you a very healthy pick-me-up, getting you back on track while improving your health and well-being.

Four Reasons You Need Morning Juice

While it's important for all of us to juice regularly to ensure we get our daily dose of fruit and veggies, if you are someone who has any of the following signs it's due time to make a valuable change—more so than just your weight loss goals:

1. *You're Tired, Lethargic and Foggy-Headed.*

   This is the worst feeling, especially when we have work to do. We don't have time to feel like crap—ever—so getting out of this funk is significant. If you're feeling knockout tired a reboot with morning juice is a great way to enhance your energy levels. By day two that foggy head should begin to clear, if not sooner.

2. *Digestive Upsets.*

   No one in the world likes to experience stomach discomfort or reflux, constipation, diarrhea or flatulence but when we pack in processed foods or quick-eats, it's not uncommon to feel all of the above quite regularly. Whipping up a morning juice will not only give your digestive system a break, it will dramatically improve digestion, aiding in weight loss.

3. *Excess Weight & Difficult/Sluggish Weight Loss.*

You're reading this book because you're ready to make a change and lose weight. Your body will thank you when you give it an unexpected nutrient and antioxidant push combined with a decrease in calories. Adding some morning juice will kick-start your weight loss journey by readjusting your palate and reducing your cravings for those no-no's, leading to weight loss success.

4. *Headache Central.*

Headaches, we all get them. But if you're someone who gets frequent headaches that is a definite sign that you're in need of a rock-solid reboot and a morning kick-off with fruits and veggies. Headaches can be caused by processed foods, poor nutrition, dehydration and a lack of sleep, so this morning juice regimen and newfound healthy diet will greatly reduce—if not eliminate—your headaches.

While there are quite a few other things that would indicate a need for a morning juicing regimen, the truth is—juicing is one of the best ways to jumpstart your weight loss journey. Juicing is perfectly paired with tossing out processed foods and executing those mini workouts.

'So, what goes in these juice blends anyway?' That's a question I hear all the time. I could go on and on, saying that

they are tasty this, really good that, but the best way for you to judge the *'Two Minute Morning Juice'* is to try it out yourself.

That said, I've concocted a handful of morning juice recipes that are not only my favorite, they are ideal for beginner juice blenders like you. These refreshing and tasty blends will take less than a minute to prepare and if you're short on time, you can always prep your blender or NutriBullet in advance.

Tasty Juice Blender Recipes for Weight Loss

Recipe One: An Orange New You

Orange juice has always been a favorite for breakfast, but orange juice doesn't necessarily have to contain oranges.

This sucker is packed with goodness and the juice is blended up with carrots, ginger, lemon and pears, adding the perfect about of sweet. Carrots provide a much higher dose of nutrients, more so than *any* type of store-bought morning juice.

Ingredients

- 8 Medium Carrots
- 1 Lemon
- 1 Pear
- .5 to 1-inch Piece of Ginger
- Handful of Baby Spinach (optional)

Directions

1. Wash all of the produce well—preferably the night before if you're in an early morning time crunch.

2. Peel the lemon. Add all ingredients to blender, juicer *or* NutriBullet. Enjoy!

Recipe Two: Summer Lovin' (Even in Winter)

I personally think *Summer Lovin'* tastes just as good (if not better) than PowerAde or Gatorade. It's refreshing in the heat of summer and brings back the taste of summer during winter.

This bad boy is packed with a healthy dose of carbohydrates, B-vitamins for energy, natural sodium and sugar, giving you an unbeatable dose of *wow!* Perfect for a morning boost or afternoon pick-me-up.

Ingredients

- ¼ Cup Pineapple
- ¼ Cup Watermelon (rind included)
- 2 Carrots
- 2 Stalks of Celery
- 1-inch Slice of Ginger

Directions

1. Wash all of the produce well—preferably the night before if you're in an early morning time crunch.

2. Peel the pineapple, cutting it into thick slices. Measure out ¼ cup, discarding the rind.

3. Add all ingredients to your blender, juicer or NutriBullet and blend for 30 seconds to 1 minute, until smooth. Pour into your preferred cup or glass and enjoy.

With the above recipe you can substitute pineapple with mango, watermelon with cantaloupe or other melon of your preference. If you don't have any carrots on hand or want to change it up a bit, butternut squash chunks or a sweet potato will add the perfect amount of sweet.

You can also add lemon or lime in place of ginger, though ginger is perfect for its natural anti-inflammatory ingredients.

Recipe Three: Brain Boost Smoothie for a Hectic Day

This recipe is perfect for the days that you simply do not feel up to par. Maybe you're just getting over a cold or just need something to get you out of that funk, this brain boosting smoothie is sure to get you through even the toughest of days. This smoothie recipe is not only brain-healthy; its taste is out of this world.

Ingredients

- 5 to 6 Strawberries
- 1 Handful of Baby Spinach
- 1 Handful Kale
- 2 Tablespoons Cacao Nibs

- Dash of Cinnamon
- Dash of Turmeric
- 8 Ounces of Almond Milk (any milk alternative will do)
- 1 Scoop Protein Powder of Choice

Directions

1. Produce and all ingredients can be prepared the night before, if on a time crunch.

2. Wash produce and prepare ingredients.

3. Add all ingredients to blender or Nutribullet and blend for approximately 60 seconds or until smooth. Pour into your glass of choice and enjoy!

There are a wide variety of smoothie and morning juice recipes readily available online, most of which are equally as good as the few mentioned above.

A morning juice routine will really help you *kick out* the bad food from your life, ridding your body of unhealthy toxins that continuously prevent you from losing the weight you've been trying to shed.

And what's great is that you can essentially pack in all this goodness in under two minutes, every single day!

If you find that the morning is one of the most hectic times in your day, you can prep your juice or smoothie recipes the night before, placing everything in your blender, ready for use. That way you can wake up, get ready for your day and throw the blender on just before rushing out to the office.

In the next chapter we are going to go into eating habits, what works, what doesn't and what's essential to pack in on your weight loss journey.

Others who are considering purchasing this book would love to know what you think. If you could spare a few seconds, they would greatly appreciate reading an honest review from you. Simply visit the page on Amazon.com.

Chapter Five

Eating Habits & Dietary Options

It's not like you were born yesterday, so you know that not all calories are created equal. There are calories that are packed full of bad fats and healthy fats, all coming from a variety of different foods. But what are the best foods to eat if you want to lose weight? Sure, everyone has their own opinion but the thing is, there are certain foods that shed those pounds faster than others.

While there are "diets" that claim to be the best—Atkins, Weight Watchers, Jenny Craig, Raw Food Diets, to name a few—but it's not a label that's going to help you lose weight. It's about what you put into your body. It's your daily eating habits and dietary choices that can make you or break you.

There are quite a few ways that you can lose weight, but what about losing weight *fast*? As human beings, we like speedy results and after years of testing and working with my friends, family and clients, I've found that what makes a world of difference (with the speed of weight loss) is a high protein, low fat and minimally processed diet packed full of good fats, greens and root vegetables.

This weeds out other carbs and starches, but despite the many claims that one should toss potatoes out of their diet, potatoes (sweet potatoes and other root veggies included) are actually the perfect food for weight loss and health.

In fact, potatoes contain a wide range of nutrients, so much so that there have been claims of people living on nothing but potatoes for an extended period of time.

Potatoes are packed full of potassium (more potassium than even bananas or spinach), vitamin C and B 6, in addition to magnesium, iron and zinc. Another plus about potatoes is that by eating boiled potatoes you will feel full and eat less of other foods.

The same goes for high protein diets as they keep you full for longer, making it less likely for you to grab snacks or sweets.

My recommended weight loss and diet plan showcased within this chapter will not only reduce your appetite quite significantly, it will ensure that you shed pounds quickly, without you 'starving to death' or hating every moment of your life (like so many other diets create).

Not only that, the ultimate goal here is also for you to improve your overall health so that you can enjoy your life to the fullest. After all, life is more than just work, work, work and once you start to feel healthier you will have more energy to fit *everything* into your schedule.

Say what? Yes, it's true.

My recommendation is to implement three *main* dietary options; changes that—when combined with your mini-workouts and morning juice regimen—will knock off those pounds in no time.

Three Dietary Options for a Healthy Life

1. *Kick Carbs and Sugar to the Curb*

Knock out or at least cut back more than ½ of your daily sugar and starch/carb intake. The main reason for this is because sugars and carbs fuel the secretion of insulin more than any other food—and insulin is a major (the main) fat storage hormone in the body.

What this means is that when your insulin level goes down, fat has an easier time getting out of the fat supplies and your body will start burning fats instead of carbs. And this! This is what we want.

Another perk of keeping your insulin level low is that low insulin levels also reduce bloat and unnecessary water weight. The reason for this is because your kidneys will have the ability to shed excess sodium and water due to the fact that they won't need to work as hard to break down sugars.

By cutting out carbs and sugars you could lose up to ten pounds within your first week (if not more). Not only will you be eating fewer calories, you eat mindlessly because you won't be hungry.

2. *Eat More Veggies & Protein.*

No matter if it's breakfast, lunch or dinner, every single one of those meals should include a protein source, healthy fats and low-carb veggies. If you're drinking your breakfast (two-minute juice), simply add a scoop of your favorite protein powder.

Vegan protein powder will keep the sugar out.*

When you opt for traditional protein for your lunch and dinner meals, it's always best to choose lean meats and other protein sources.

Healthy protein sources include:

- o Beef, Chicken, Pork, Lamb, Turkey Bacon
- o Salmon, Trout, Shrimp, Tilapia
- o Eggs (omega-3 enriched, free range eggs are best)

There's no reason to skimp on protein. A high-protein intake can boost your metabolism greatly, making it that much easier to shed the pounds. Not only that, it's been proven that having a high protein diet **reduces obsessive thoughts about food** by more than 60%!

So, what about veggies?

Sticking to low-carb veggies such as spinach, kale, brussel sprouts, cabbage, cauliflower, celery, Swiss chard, broccoli and lettuce is essential. These vegetables are packed full of nutrients and because they are low-carb you can eat as much as you want. Load up, veggies are good!

Keeping your diet focused on protein, vegetable and minimal fat will help you lose weight in no time. Good fats can come from olive oil, coconut oil, avocado oil (and avocados) and butter.

Try to make sure that you eat at least two to three meals each day. And with each meal it's important to include a protein option, vegetable and healthy fat. For your morning shake/juice, an avocado slice is the perfect healthy fat addition.

3. Mini-Workouts and You.

While mini-workouts and exercise is not a dietary option, daily exercise plays a crucial role to weight loss. Sure, you can lose weight without exercise if you follow the two dietary options listed above, but exercise will help you lose weight faster.

These mini-workouts will burn calories and prevent your metabolism from slowing down—a common side effect of losing weight.

There have been quite a few studies that show a high-protein, low-carb diet is the best option to lose a significant amount of body fat, regardless of whether it's 5 pounds you're looking to lose or 100 pounds.

This life reboot might seem like a lot to consider, especially making all these changes at once, but with a low-carb, high-protein diet you can essentially eat anything you want including your favorite foods and even your favorite recipes, with a few modifications.

A Body Re-Feed

Unfortunately, part of losing weight is the natural *want* for what we can't—or shouldn't have. It's only normal for this *want* to weigh in a frustrate us once in a while, and this is one reason why it's completely okay to give yourself one day off each week or every other week.

Not everyone wants to utilize this freebie, but it's not uncommon for a day off to make your newfound routine that much easier.

This doesn't mean that you completely take advantage of that day off and binge eat food that's bad for you. It just means that you can enjoy one of your favorite snacks one day out of the week—in moderation, of course.

For instance, let's say you've been really good about bringing a healthy alternative to the movie theater instead of your favorite movie-theater popcorn. Well, let yourself go one or two days out of the month. It's completely okay if you keep up with your high-protein, low-carb diet on all other days.

Make Saturday or Sunday your off day, giving yourself a break. Keep in mind, however, that you can only give yourself **one allotment.**

If you start slacking and having multiple cheat meals per week you won't see much success, and shedding those pounds will take much longer than it should.

Keep in mind that giving yourself a cheat meal isn't necessary. If you feel 100% okay with your new day-to-day routine, stick with it.

That Thing Called Portion Control

We've heard that eating smaller portions will help us lose weight a million and one times, right? Maybe that's true if you're eating anything and everything, making a minimal change to your diet, but if you're sticking with a high-protein, healthy fat and low-carb diet (packed with veggies), you won't need to count calories.

By sticking to the plan mentioned within this chapter and throughout my book, you'll lose your first few pounds in no time—most likely within the first couple of days!

If you keep your carb intake to approximately 20-50 grams, you'll shed pounds fast and keep them off.

Five Tips to Lose Weight Even Faster!

The reason I love the routine and diet mentioned in this book is because *it works*...and works fast. But we all know that patience can be difficult and *fast* just might not be *fast enough*.

The following five tips will make your weight loss journey easier and will also help you shed those pounds faster, so that you can live as a happier and healthier new you:

1. *High Protein Mornings*

Pack in the protein each morning to reduce cravings throughout the day. As mentioned earlier, adding a protein powder to your two-minute morning juice will suffice.

However, if you decide to skip the morning juice a day or two, free-range eggs with turkey bacon or sausage and boiled potatoes would be a great alternative. This will keep you full until lunch (if not longer).

2. *Drink Cold Water ½ Hour Before Meals*

Down that 8-ounce glass of water thirty minutes before meals to speed up your weight loss. A recent study showed that drinking water drinking cold water before each meal will increase your weight loss by 44%!

3. *Avoid Sugar-Filled Drinks (including Fruit Juice)*

Sugary drinks and fruit juice are essentially like drinking your weight. While fruit juice might have vitamin C, the calories and sugar can really put a damper on your diet. Not only that, additional sugar can make you sluggish.

4. Choose Fresh Produce & Lean Meats

Say goodbye to processed foods. They might taste good, but after ridding your body of processed foods, you'll realize that it was your mind that tricked you into thinking these things were good.

Sticking with high-protein from lean meats and fresh produce will keep you on the right track. Whole foods also keep you filled up faster, making it that much more likely that you won't grab an unhealthy alternative for an afternoon snack.

5. Soluble Fiber is Your Friend

Fiber supplements are proven to aid in weight loss, reducing fat, especially in the belly area. In fact, a recent study showed that glucomannan is the only dietary fiber known to cause modest weight loss when taken as a daily supplement.

Sticking with these five tips will help you lose weight faster. It's also recommended that you eat your food slower and use smaller plates. Eating slowly will put less strain on your digestive system and you will tend to feel full, faster.

All in all, if you follow this entire dietary plan, including mini-workouts, you can expect to lose at least five to ten pounds in your first week. This weight loss should stay consistent if you stick with the plan. I've lost 3-5 pounds per week consistently when I follow this regimen.

Keep in mind that since you're suddenly switching your food intake and what your body is used to 'thriving' on, it's not uncommon to experience what I like to call the low-carb flu. You might feel like you're in a fog and not your normal spunky self, but it will pass—usually by day three.

During the first three days you might be tempted to load up on carbs to feel better, but this flu passes quickly and the weight loss that you will experience within the first week is well worth those few days of yuck.

Love Yourself, Don't Starve Yourself

As with any change in diet or routine, it's recommended to talk to your doctor before making any dramatic changes. If you have a medical condition, this plan could potentially reduce your need for recommendation and it might be something your doctor will recommend after weekly monitoring of your condition and/or weight loss.

There's no reason for you to go into a diet plan and starve yourself with the hope that you will lose weight faster. In most cases, this never happens because your body stores fat for later use (in the case that we cannot eat).

By reducing your carb intake, you will dramatically reduce your appetite and hunger, eliminating the main reason people fail with conventional weight loss methods.

With my method showcased throughout this book, you will be able to lose weight faster and keep it off due to the fact that you're adjusting your life and routine, promoting a healthier, happier you.

In fact, I've tried and tested this approach time and time again, and found that I've actually lost more than three times as much weight as I did on a low-fat or calorie restricted diet. And with this high-protein low-carb diet I can basically eat all the good food I want until I'm full yet still shed pounds regularly.

Can't beat that, right?

Within the next closing chapter, I'm going to discuss the importance of weekend planning. Planning and even prepping your meals every weekend can make sticking to this new diet that much easier due to the fact that it will ensure you eat these high-protein, veggie packed alternatives rather than loading up on carbs and processed food (due to the lack of time in your day).

I hope you have learned something from this book so far and would greatly appreciate it if you could leave an honest review on Amazon.com.

Chapter Six

Weekend Meal Prep for Success

It's no secret that people prep their weekly meals on the weekend, but you might be asking yourself, *'Does this really make a difference?'* The simple answer is yes.

There are many reasons why the weekend meal prep is essential including:

1. You become less tempted to cheat.
2. Saves you money on groceries (and eating out each week).
3. Saves on time, especially for the business professional like yourself or stay-at-home mom.
4. Helps you meet your fitness goals.
5. You're never bored with food options!

All of this sounds great, right? Looking at this list you can probably see why meal prep is a precursor to weight loss success—especially number one.

If you already have your meals planned out and keep processed food out of your life, you won't have any temptation to cheat and grab something easy.

What I recommend is writing out your weekly grocery list on Friday or Saturday, shopping for all things on that list (no extras!), and calling it a day.

Doing this will not only save you tons of money, you will be less tempted because you won't have any additional junk in your cabinets. So, one and two go hand-in-hand.

Now, one of my favorite perks of the weekend meal prep is saving time! And if you're reading this book, this one is for you.

Not only will meal prepping keep us on track with our diet, it gives us more time throughout the week to get in mini-workouts or family fitness in the evenings.

I mean let's be honest, with rush-hour and sitting in traffic after working a 9 to 5 job or carting around the children, it's overwhelming to think about getting in exercise or having enough time to make dinner.

By preparing our meals in advanced, we simply pull them out of the fridge or freezer, nuke them in the microwave or oven, and we are good to go!

And what we are feeding our mind and body is all healthy, whole foods—exactly what we need to stay on track with our diet.

While it might be true that meal prep can feel a little monotonous, there are so many different recipes available online that will keep your meal prep interesting and tasty.

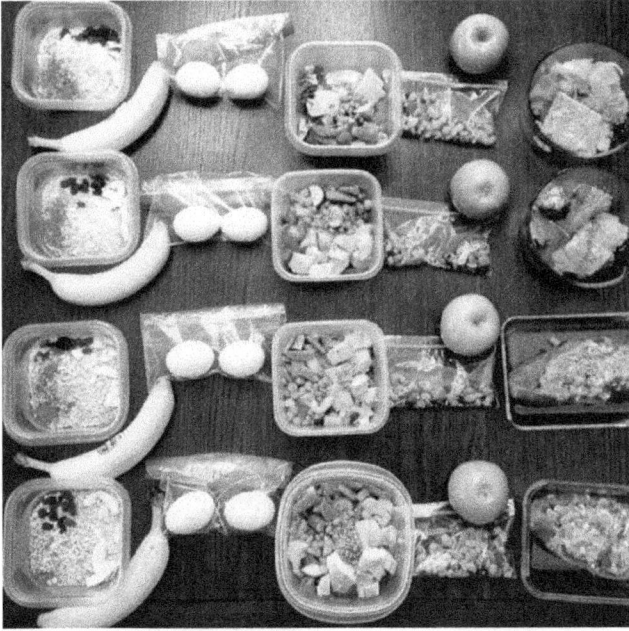

For instance, say you're planning on making chicken breast for the week but really don't want to be eating the same flavors day in and day out. Who does?!

But by utilizing aluminum foil as dividers and a large baking pan, you can cook three to four different types of chicken at one time—BBQ chicken, blacked chicken, honey mustard, you name it.

Another trick for easy prep is to freeze your morning juice or smoothie in muffin tins. All you need to do is buy your two-minute juice ingredients in bulk, whip up your favorite recipes on the weekend and toss them in a muffin tin to freeze.

Once frozen, you can simply toss two or three of these smoothie cups into the blender and run!

This makes breakfast a breeze and overall it shouldn't take you more than 30 minutes on the weekend to prep the juice blends and add them to a muffin tin for freezing.

Vegetables stay for a long time in the fridge once chopped and prepped for use, at least 5 days. This means that you can prep your veggies for the week, including zucchini noodles or 'Zoodles' (perfect replacement for pasta!) and butternut squash, and seal them in containers. You can use zucchini for lasagna, spaghetti and meatballs and more.

And no, you don't have to give up cheese!

See? You can have all of your favorite foods with minor modifications. Losing weight doesn't mean that you need to give up your happiness and things you enjoy. It is all about moderation, being conscious of what you're consuming and how you prep your food.

Before you set off to the grocery store and shop for your week of groceries it's important that you invest in some quality containers. It doesn't matter if they are glass or plastic, but since you will be re-heating your food for meals it's wise to choose containers that are BPA-free and won't fall apart in the microwave.

If you plan on putting your prepped meal in the oven to heat-through, grab oven-safe glass wear so that you don't have to dirty more dishes. These days, most oven-safe containers come with a lid, making it easy to keep meal preps fresh for the week.

For your first meal-prep week I actually recommend setting aside a couple days for the task. Once you get used to the process it's likely that you can prep everything in a day, but when you're just getting started it might wise to set aside a couple days for cooking.

The last thing you want is to become overwhelmed and discouraged. Keep in mind that cooking for the week is a big deal, especially if you're cooking for a family. At first it might feel like you're preparing a Thanksgiving feast, but taking things slow and keeping things simple will minimize stress.

This new routine and life you're creating is exciting, especially because you know that you're going to be successful on this weight loss journey. There's nothing holding you back except yourself, but my hope is that after reading this book you're ready for this mission—both mentally and physically.

You've got this. This is your time to shine.

Don't forget to share your thoughts on this book by leaving a review on Amazon.com. It takes just a few seconds.

Discover Scientifically-Proven "Shortcuts" & "Hacks" to Lose Weight FASTER (With Very Little Effort)

For this month only, you can get Linda's best-selling & most popular book absolutely free – *Weight Loss Secrets You NEED to Know*.

Get Your FREE Copy Here:

TopFitnessAdvice.com/Bonus

Discover scientifically-proven tips to help you lose weight faster and easier than ever before. With this book, readers were able to improve their weight loss results and fitness levels. So, it's highly recommended that you get this book, especially while it's free!

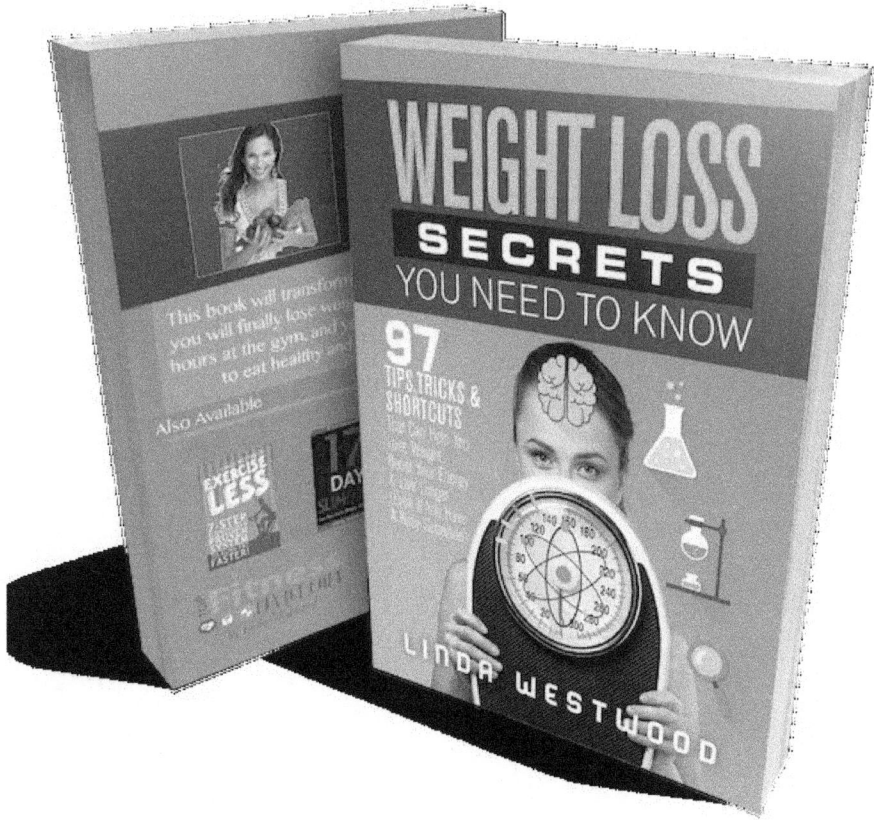

Get Your FREE Copy Here:

TopFitnessAdvice.com/Bonus

Conclusion

I hope that by reading this book you're ready and motivated about the future. By implementing the tips I have given you throughout this book, you will not only dramatically improve your overall health and wellness, you will also experience a boost in self-esteem when you realize that **you can do anything you put your mind to**.

Sure, your schedule is hectic and jam-packed with meetings, soccer games or ballet recitals, but being busy is not who you are. You're an incredible person who can essentially have anything they want. Yes, this includes losing that ten to twenty pounds that you've wanted to lose for the last five to ten years.

Remember, the first battle to conquer is your mindset and once you live in the moment and push aside doubt and negativity, your life—as a whole—will begin to transform.

The key to a successful change of routine is a positive mindset or a switch in limited thinking. When we are wrapped up in our current life or situation, we often think that there's *no possible way* to make a change, especially if it requires some *more* of your time. I mean, you barely have enough time to breathe, how on Earth could you exercise or make a home cooked meal?

As we learned, your mindset, good, healthy eats, lots of protein and veggies, low-carbs, mini-workouts and meal prep will make a enormous difference in your everyday life. If you keep with the routine you *will* lose five to ten pounds in the first week, and at least three to five pounds every week after until you're at your desired weight.

Once you have reached your weight loss goal, you will be astonished to find that this routine that you are creating is one that will last and become a way of life, even for the busiest of people.

Somehow between the hustle and bustle of everyday life, all that's required of you at the office or at home with your children and significant other, you will suddenly have the time to make all of your dreams come true. Better yet, you will also find that your quality of life dramatically increases, creating a happier, more fulfilled, healthier you.

Final Words

I would like to thank you for purchasing my book and I hope I have been able to help you and educate you on something new.

If you have enjoyed this book and would like to share your positive thoughts, could you please take 30 seconds of your time to go back and give me a review on my Amazon book page.

I greatly appreciate seeing these reviews because it helps me share my hard work.

You can leave me a review on Amazon.com.

Again, thank you and I wish you all the best!

Enjoying this book?

Check out my other best sellers!

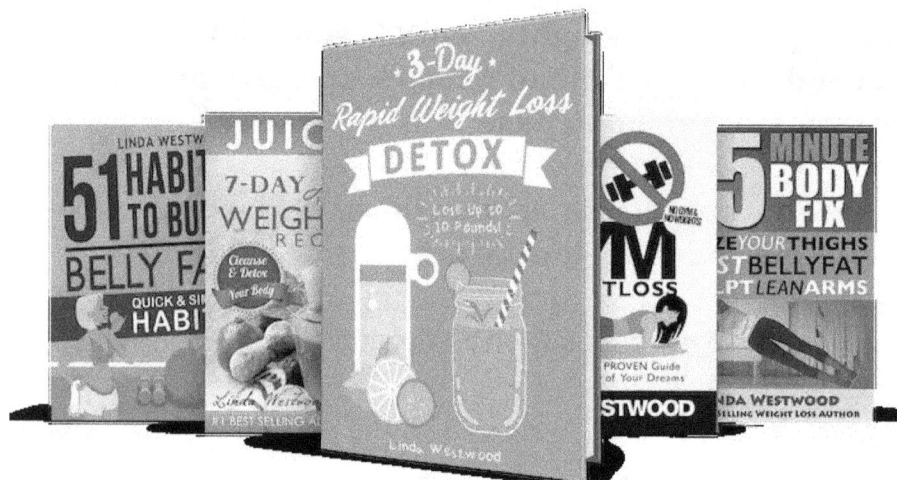

www.ingramcontent.com/pod-product-compliance
Lightning Source LLC
Chambersburg PA
CBHW031205020426
42333CB00013B/804